# HOW TO PERSUADE YOUR LOVER TO USE A CONDOM
## ... AND WHY YOU SHOULD

# HOW TO PERSUADE YOUR LOVER TO USE A CONDOM ... AND WHY YOU SHOULD

PATTI BREITMAN
KIM KNUTSON
PAUL REED

PRODUCED BY
NEW YORK PUBLISHING
SAN FRANCISCO, CALIFORNIA

PRIMA PUBLISHING AND COMMUNICATIONS
Post Office Box 1260PC
Rocklin, California 95677

**READER PLEASE NOTE:** Condoms are not 100 percent effective in either the prevention of pregnancy or the prevention of sexually transmitted disease. The only foolproof way to prevent pregnancy or sexually transmitted disease is abstinence or no-risk sex, such as masturbation. With proper condom use, however, one can reduce the chances of unplanned pregnancy or infection of sexually transmitted disease. There are many forms of birth control and options for disease prevention. Questions asked about individual sexual behaviors and their associated risks should be addressed to your physician. Your doctor can advise you about risk factors and appropriate methods for risk reduction, of which condom use may be one.

Produced by NEW YORK PUBLISHING, San Francisco
Cover design by Dunlavey Studio
Typography by *turnaround*, Berkeley

Prima Publishing & Communications
P.O. Box 1260PC
Rocklin, CA 95677
(916) 624-5718

Library of Congress Cataloging-in-Publication Data
Breitman, Patti, 1954–
How to persuade your lover to use a condom.
Resource Directory: p.
1. Hygiene, Sexual. 2. Condoms. I. Knutson, Kim, 1961–
II. Reed, Paul, 1956–
III. Title.
RA788.B727   1987          6713.9'5          86–30186
ISBN 0-914629-43-3

10  9  8  7  6  5  4  3  2  1
87  88  89  90  91
Printed in the United States of America

# CONTENTS

# FOREWORD

*by*

**John Money, Ph.D.**

*Professor of Medical Psychology and
Professor of Pediatrics, Emeritus
The Johns Hopkins University and Hospital
Baltimore, Maryland*

When I first learned about condoms from my cousin—
he was fifteen, I was thirteen—they were "rubbers,"
and it was daring and adventurous to use them. It was
also erotic and grown-up—and loads of fun. They were
fun to masturbate with and, later in my teens, fun for a
partner and me to play with together in preparation for
sexual intercourse. Sure, they were joked about as raincoats. For a teenaged couple, however, condoms were
the only way to have sex without getting pregnant or
catching venereal disease (VD).

VD was still a terrifying scourge when I was seven-
teen. That was in 1938. I was a freshman undergraduate
majoring in psychology, and I spent the summer working in the medical ward of the state mental hospital. I
still remember the coagulated eyeballs of a once famous
cello player as he wasted away, blind and demented,
from tabes dorsalis, the third and final stage of syphilis.
I used to wonder how often he and others with the
same fate asked themselves, "Why didn't I use a condom?" There was, in that era before penicillin, no cure

for syphilis or gonorrhea. In fact it would not be until 1947, when I left New Zealand for the United States, that penicillin came on the market. It ushered in an era of sexual freedom devoid of the horrors of syphilis and gonorrhea.

Penicillin attacks bacterial infections but not viruses. It gives no protection against the sexually transmitted herpes virus which, although nothing new, grabbed the headlines in the late 1970s. The best protection against catching the genital herpes virus from a contagious partner is to have the protection of a condom. The penalty of exposure is not lethal, except possibly to a baby being delivered by a mother with herpes.

The VD wheel, having changed its name to sexually transmitted disease (STD) has done a full turn and now is stuck at acquired immune deficiency syndrome (AIDS). This disease, caused by the new virus, human immunodeficiency virus (HIV) is more lethal than syphilis and more horrendous in the torture with which it kills you. AIDS can kill as soon as six months or as late as several years after the virus invades the bloodstream. The longest survival time after becoming infected is not yet known. One way of becoming infected is from a needle contaminated (even invisibly) with blood from someone who already has the virus. The other way of becoming infected is by taking into one's own body the sexual fluids of a partner who has the virus. (There is as yet no final answer as to how much risk there is in tongue kissing a person who has the AIDS virus.)

Getting the AIDS virus into the penis, vagina, rectum, or mouth is almost as risky as playing Russian roulette with all the barrels loaded. There is no guaranteed 100% effective safeguard, but the best safeguard available, for women and men, gay and straight, is a condom. AIDS kills anyone it can get in its clutches: man, woman, or child; homosexual, bisexual, or heterosexual. Anyone with whom you have sex who has had sex with someone other than yourself in the past few days, weeks, months, or years is a potential carrier of the virus. That is why AIDS is spreading so fast, among women as well as men, and why it is truly an epidemic. There is still no cure. Prevention is what counts.

Whether you are gay or straight, the first act of prevention is persuading yourself not to be sexually penetrated unless your lover uses a condom and not to sexually penetrate unless you use one. The only person for whom you can be fully responsible is yourself. Teaching, preaching, and judging usually fall on deaf ears.

A saying that I've quoted innumerable times is this: for effective communication, *don't teach, preach, or judge. Just tell.* Always tell about yourself—your present thoughts, feelings, and convictions, and your predictions about what they will be if such-and-such happens. Begin every sentence with *I.* It sounds easy, but it actually requires a bit of practice, for our language is ordinarily full of teaching, preaching, and judging.

One way to avoid these pitfalls is to begin conversing about a topic that belongs in the public domain—something that everybody knows about. For example: "I saw the TV special on AIDS last weekend, and it scared me to death. Can we talk about it?" Such an opening gambit is likely to get your partner talking about the AIDS scare also, and before long you might both be discussing the pros and cons of sex with a condom.

If biomedical science finally conquers this disease, there will no longer be a terrible penalty for not using a condom. Today the penalty is so great that common sense says, "Never be without one and use one every time!"

This is a message that should be on TV for all ages, to be learned when young and put into practice when one begins sexual activity. It should be a strong message, demonstrating without prudery or silliness how to be a couple who together enjoy the normal and healthy pleasures of sex while using a condom.

# PART ONE
# SEX TODAY

If you believe that a good sex life is your right, and you aren't willing to choose abstinence when there are other options, then this book is for you. It will reassure you, help you feel comfortable with condoms, and help you persuade your partner to use them.

We wrote this book because we're angry. All the magazine articles and newspaper stories about AIDS are telling us to use condoms. Even the Surgeon General is urging us to use them, but no one is addressing the simple fact that *people don't like condoms.*

If you are divorced, you're probably facing your new dating situation with some serious doubts and questions about the risks of sexual intimacy. If you're single, maybe you've begun to think about a permanent relationship with someone as a safer lifestyle. If you're gay, you've been aware of the AIDS risk longer than most others, and you have probably made some difficult decisions regarding your own sex life.

These are our exact situations. Patti, who is from New York, is divorced and in her early thirties. Kim, who grew up in North Dakota, is in her mid-twenties and single. Paul, also in his early thirties, is a native Californian. He's gay and has been in a steady relationship during the last several years.

Among our friends are happily married people who are worried about their pasts, unhappy couples who are afraid to leave the sexual safety of their relationships, women who have had unwanted pregnancies, men and women who have chosen celibacy over intimacy because of fear. We have lost friends to AIDS, and we have friends who have been infected with the AIDS virus and who live with the anxiety of uncertainty about their own futures.

The best way to approach sex today is not with anxiety and fear, but by looking at the facts and making positive choices about how we live our lives.

Some of those facts can be frightening, but we don't want to scare you with this book. We intentionally toned down our passionate arguments to try to counteract the panic that news stories have stirred up—and to show you how to argue with a reluctant partner calmly yet insistently, with facts not terror.

But *do* be passionate in your argument. Use whatever reasons, strategies, and facts you can to convince your lover that condoms are the right choice for both of you. Be patient, but be firm. And know that you are not alone.


## CONDOMS TODAY

Condoms, rubbers, prophylactics, balloons, sheaths,

safes, skins, white fish, raincoats, protection. Condoms have many names. They also have many reputations. Some people think condoms are used only by prostitutes to keep them from getting venereal diseases. Others believe condoms are a symbol of the playboy always ready for sex. Some people are embarrassed to keep condoms handy.

Even people who don't think of condoms as dirty often still don't like to use them. They think that condoms are for fumbling teenagers or that condoms are a big turn-off. Some men find them uncomfortable to wear. Some men and some women complain that they miss skin contact during intercourse. Others say that putting on a condom interrupts the excitement of sex. And then there's the expression that "making love with a condom is like wearing a raincoat in the shower."

Condoms were out of style in the United States for a long time. Other forms of birth control made condoms seem clumsy and inconvenient, and the widespread availability of antibiotics lessened the threat of most sexually transmitted diseases. But today many people want to use condoms again, because condoms are an effective form of birth control and, more important, because they are effective in disease prevention.

Condoms have been around for centuries. Long before we had latex and modern manufacturing, people used animal membranes as sheaths for the penis. Today condoms are still used throughout the world. More condoms are used in Japan than in any other country, in part because the Japanese have never legalized birth control pills. Americans buy 800,000 condoms a day, and recent studies show that there is an upward trend in condom sales (reported in *Fortune*, November 26, 1986).

Today condoms are the focus of much media attention and debate. Condom manufacturers are developing new brands. Public health departments are issuing brochures giving information about condoms. And the public is looking for answers to many questions about condoms and their proper use.

## THE THREAT OF AIDS

The threat of AIDS has made condoms important again. Dissatisfaction with other forms of birth control is also playing a part in many people's decision to use condoms. But it is the threat of AIDS that is most strongly influencing the public to use condoms. Public health officials worldwide are urging people to use condoms to avoid the spread of the AIDS virus.

It is a serious situation, and the facts about AIDS are not as widely known as they ought to be. Because the AIDS epidemic spread through the gay community *first*, the media reported the situation in such a way that heterosexual people were given a false sense of security—AIDS was something that happened to somebody else. As a result, a dangerous situation has arisen, because people who are at risk may believe that they are not.

From the beginning of the AIDS epidemic in 1981, a proportion of people getting sick were *not* gay. These were people who contracted the disease through sharing contaminated needles during intravenous drug use, through receiving transfusions of infected blood, or in other ways—including transmission during heterosexual sex. That proportion has grown over the years, and the need is now greater than ever for all of us to recognize AIDS as a serious threat to everyone. The need is urgent to educate the entire public about measures it can take to lower the risk of infection.

The need is *urgent* because of the silent way the AIDS virus spreads. Being infected with the AIDS virus is not the same thing as having the full-blown disease. Not everyone who becomes infected with the virus goes on to develop the full disease, but among those who do, the length of time it takes to develop full-blown AIDS can be from a few months to *many years.* Throughout that period of infection, an individual may have no symptoms whatsoever—in fact, most infected people don't—and may not even suspect that he or she has been infected. Such a person can unknowingly infect others.

That's why we're seeing so many new cases of the fully developed disease as time goes on: some people were infected many years ago—many before anyone even knew about it. Although AIDS was first recognized in 1981, scientists didn't understand just how it was spread until 1983, when the virus was isolated and identified. Yet the cases identified in 1981 probably resulted from infection dating to the late 1970s.

## WHY CONDOMS ARE IMPORTANT IN PREVENTING AIDS

Because of this long incubation period for AIDS, and because so many people are infected without knowing it, it is important to take action *now* to prevent cases of AIDS that could appear years from now. This is where condoms are important in prevention. The experience that the gay community has had with AIDS since 1981 offers insight into the steps that can be taken to combat the disease.

As soon as doctors explained just how the AIDS virus was transmitted, the gay community began a massive campaign to slow the spread of new infection. This campaign includes widespread education about condom use, safe sexual practices, health and hygiene, and stress reduction. This campaign is working to slow the spread of new AIDS infection and to lessen the occurrence of other sexually transmitted diseases. In cities with large gay populations, studies have shown that the rate of new AIDS infection has dropped within the gay community and the overall rate of occurrence of gonorrhea and syphilis has dropped significantly.

That means that *education as a preventive measure works*—education about condoms and safe sex. But the AIDS virus continues to spread increasingly among other groups of people, including heterosexuals.

# WHY CONDOMS ARE IMPORTANT AS A METHOD OF BIRTH CONTROL

As people become increasingly concerned about the relative safety of various forms of birth control, the condom is receiving renewed attention as a simple option. Condom use does not require the taking of medication or the use of invasive apparatus. And when used in conjunction with a spermicidal jelly, condoms are highly effective as a birth control method.

But most important, the advantage that condoms have as a method of birth control is that they also provide protection from sexually transmitted disease.

# THE DEBATE ABOUT CONDOMS

Whenever there is a need to bring sensitive information to the public, there is debate about appropriateness, tastefulness, and the moral issues involved. The issue of birth control arouses debate based on religious beliefs and moral values, and the issue of sexual behavior as related to disease is complex and confusing.

Because this is a serious situation requiring everybody's cooperation, the feelings of all people must be considered. But forming public policy takes time. The life-threatening nature of the AIDS epidemic makes the need to do something about it urgent. The conflict between the need to form a balanced public policy and the need to take immediate action intensifies the emotions surrounding the debate.

Because of the experience the gay community has had in dealing with AIDS, the straight community need not go through *all* the debates that the gay community has successfully resolved. We don't have to view AIDS as something about which we don't know what to do. If the straight community will adopt the kind of campaign for prevention through education that has worked in the gay community, it will be possible to save many, many lives.

There is no time to waste. We must listen to all arguments, but while the debate goes on, we must take immediate action to slow the spread of new infection. One of the things people can do right away is use condoms during sex.

## IS THIS BOOK FOR YOU?

We wrote this book for all kinds of people, because we believe that using condoms is important for all sexually active people—male or female, straight or gay, young or old. Whether you are single and dating, in a relationship, or married, this book contains valuable information about condoms—how to use them and how to persuade your sex partner to use them.

People vary in their sexual activities, and this book takes that fact into account. Something that might seem complicated to you might seem simple to someone else; something that might seem strange to you might be another's common practice. So please keep in mind that we have written for a wide audience.

## A NEW SEXUAL AWARENESS

Sex is a uniquely wonderful part of life, but it is not without its responsibilities. That it carries the power to create life has long been understood, but perhaps not properly respected. Now that sex carries also the power to destroy life, we must look at sex with a new awareness, and engage in sex only after mature consideration and in a responsible way.

# PART TWO

# HOW TO
# PERSUADE
# YOUR LOVER
# TO USE
# A CONDOM

If you're going to persuade your lover to use a condom, you must be clear about the facts pertaining to your situation—whether your concern is disease, birth control, or both. In Part Three those facts are presented, and Part Four answers your questions about how to use condoms.

This section gives you advice, inspiration, and arguments you can use to persuade your lover to use a condom.

When we say "use a condom," we mean that both partners are "using" the condom for the protection of both. Obviously only men actually wear condoms, but women also benefit from the protection condoms offer.

## HOW, WHEN, AND WHERE
## TO BRING UP THE SUBJECT

Timing is important and every situation is different.

If you're single and dating, you'll want to field your potential partner's thoughts about condom use before you become sexually involved. This may require a quiet conversation or a plain negotiation in a bar before going home with someone.

Whether you are single or in a relationship, there are several ways to bring up the subject. If you already know your partner's feelings about condoms and are unhappy about them, you'll want to choose a place that is private to talk. If you don't already know how your partner feels, you might consider bringing it up when you're alone, feeling comfortable, and free of tension. Or you might bring the subject up in a general way— say, at a party or over drinks with friends—introducing condoms as a general topic of discussion.

It is difficult to know *what to say*, how to begin the conversation. Make it easier by bringing up the broader subjects connected with using a condom. You may have already discussed them—contraception (the choices) or sexually transmitted diseases (AIDS is frequently in the news).

Broach the subject with care, but be frank about your concerns, whatever they are. And remember to state them as *your* concerns, so that your partner does not feel as if he or she is under scrutiny.

Whatever approach you choose, remember to be as warm and as patient as you can. There are several opening phrases you can use to start the conversation. If you have just met someone—at a bar or party, for instance—you can start a conversation about using condoms by saying: *"This is awkward for me, but I've been thinking it would be a good idea to use condoms. What do you think?"* You could also ask him, *"Have you ever used a condom?"*

If you don't know your partner very well, but you think you will soon have sex with that person, you can be direct in your approach and try saying something like: *"I always use condoms. I always have. It just makes sense with all the things you can catch."* Or, you can bring up the subject in a positive way: *"I'd love to make it with you, but I always use condoms."*

If you've been dating the same person for a while or are in a relationship, and you are hesitant about your partner's view of condoms, you can bring up the topic generally, perhaps with others around, by saying: *"I was in the drugstore today and saw a condom display they just put up. It made me start thinking about how things are changing."* Or you might say: *"Have you seen the TV ads for condoms? I never thought I'd see something like that, but it did make me think."*

Again, if you have been dating or are in a relationship, and you want to have a private discussion, you could start by simply asking your partner: *"What do you think about using condoms?"* Another way to decrease the awkwardness is to say casually: *"I was talking with some friends the other day, and they're all using condoms now just to be careful. I think it makes a lot of sense."* If birth control is a concern, you can say: *"I've been reading that condoms are actually a very good contraceptive, with very low risk."*

In any situation you can be very honest about your fears and concerns, saying something like: *"This whole AIDS thing has got me spooked. I'm not going to give up sex, but until they find something to cure AIDS, I'm going to play it safe and insist on using condoms every time I have sex."*

Whatever you say, try to phrase it so that you leave the door open for discussion. You can do this by remembering to add a question such as, "What do you think?"

Some of these opening lines are more appropriate for people who are already dating than for people on a first date or just meeting for the first time in a bar or disco. In either case, it is important to persuade your lover to use a condom *before* you start having sex. Remember that the way you phrase your opening line and persuasive arguments is important—particularly if you are already in a relationship with someone and you want to change your sexual routine to include condoms. Reassure your partner that you are not accusing him or her of having a disease, but that you just want to be safer from now on.

Whatever your approach, don't waver in your commitment. Using condoms is a responsible way to reduce your risks of disease or unwanted pregnancy every time you have sex. But awkwardness, voiced dissatisfaction from your partner, and even manipulative complaints from your lover can be major obstacles. Remember: your self esteem and commitment to use a condom will help you overcome these obstacles. You deserve to be protected by using a condom. You deserve to feel you are making a good choice.

## IT'S NOT ALWAYS EASY

Starting this kind of conversation may be one of the hardest things you'll ever have to do. Unlike most other subjects that require serious discussion, nothing will ever be as difficult to bring up with your partner as this, because the reason *why* we need to make such an effort is so overwhelming and frightening. But once you've overcome your own objections, once you've made a commitment to use condoms, you will be ready to initiate discussion and see that you get the outcome you want— to use condoms every time.

If you find this impossible—just too difficult to do— you've got to ask yourself why. Is it your own fears? Are you unclear on the facts about AIDS? Are you worried about how your lover will react? All of these are normal and understandable concerns, but you can't let them interfere with your commitment to protect yourself. If you have unresolved feelings, perhaps you should consider not having sex until you've had some time to think it over.

In any case, it's not unusual to feel vulnerable, unsure, angry, and even silly. Becoming accustomed to using condoms and persuading your lover to use condoms is not something that happens overnight. Eventually, though, if you work at it and give yourself time, you can develop a positive attitude that will influence your lover and others to follow your example.

This is the real goal, after all—to be comfortable in being safe, to experience the reassurance that being responsible creates. Our society is uptight about sex— especially when it comes to talking about it. That's why, even with all the suggestions we've given above, it may still be enormously difficult for you to start the conversation. But you have to do it, whether it's with your steady lover or a series of different dates. We all have to reach a level of communication that allows us to talk about safe sex (see page 39 for a definition of safe sex) and about condoms without embarrassment.

Sex is nothing to be ashamed of and neither is discussing ways to protect yourself from infection or unwanted pregnancy. In fact, dealing with these concerns is a sign of wisdom and maturity.

## HOW YOU CAN REPLY
## TO ALMOST ANY RESPONSE

Once you've opened the subject for discussion, you will receive one of a number of responses. Your partner could say anything from "Great, I'd like to use condoms too" to "Never in a million years." If the response is anything other than "Yes," you need to talk more.

Be understanding. If your partner is reluctant to use condoms, try to understand why. There are a number of reasons why women and men may not want to use condoms during sex. Those reasons are usually based on feelings rather than experience. You can gently and lovingly challenge these reasons until your partner agrees with you.

Both men and women might respond with hurt feelings, shock, or anger. This is understandable, because many people are feeling the pressures of the sudden changes we're experiencing with regard to sex, disease, and birth control. Because all the new facts can be confusing, many people become frustrated. If you meet with an angry response or if your partner is utterly dismayed, stay calm. Gently remind your partner that you've given this a lot of thought, that of course you're not trying to control or force the situation, but that you would really like to talk about it.

This section presents some of the objections you might encounter when you suggest using condoms—and some answers to these objections.

*"It doesn't feel as good. I would miss the skin-to-skin contact. I just couldn't feel really intimate with a barrier between us."*

Your partner is right. The sensation that the penis feels is slightly less, but people who use condoms regularly do get used to this. And the emotional reassurance that the condom brings may more than make up for the marginal reduction in physical sensation.

This is probably the most common argument. As you get used to the feelings of sex with a condom, you can change your emotions by reminding yourself how safe you're being or by thinking of the condom as something helpful.

If a man can't adjust to the lessened physical sensation, he can try adding a drop of water-based lubricant (such as KY jelly) to the head of the penis before putting the condom on. (Never use an oil-based lubricant such as petroleum jelly; it could destroy the condom.) The lubricant will create more sensation, because it will make the end of the condom wetter and more slippery on the penis.

Ask your partner, *"I understand it will feel a little different at first, but could we try using them a few times?"* Tell your lover, *"It would make me feel safer, more relaxed. I think the difference in sensation might not seem that big after we get used to using them."*

**"I don't like to interrupt sex to put on the condom. It destroys the spontaneity."**

The idea that condoms interrupt the flow of love-making is a common complaint of both men and women. It is an inconvenience to stop what you're doing, walk to the bathroom, search through the medicine chest, walk back to the bedroom, open the package, and put on the condom.

Tell your partner you will try to make sex more spontaneous by having the condom nearby. Keep plenty of condoms available and keep them wherever you might have sex. Not only will you become accustomed to having them handy, you will be confident that you can be ready whenever and wherever you are being sexy. Condoms can become a regular part of your life, and you can get used to having them with you and handy at all times—in your backpack, purse, or briefcase; in the car or travel case; in the bedroom, bathroom, living room, and kitchen.

Just as important as having a condom available is having it ready when it's time to use it. Rather than tear open a package when you're aroused, open a package (or two or three) before the need for the condom is urgent. Put it within reach.

Try to include your partner in the act of putting the condom on. If your partner puts it on for you, it can be part of your erotic play. If you'd rather put it on yourself, face your partner and let your partner watch. What may seem clinical or even embarrassing at first can become a sexy part of lovemaking.

Say to your partner, *"I know it* can *break the sponteneity,*

*but it doesn't have to. I'll make sure condoms are close by—
and we can put it on together. At first it might be a little
disruptive, but we can practice as much as you want!"*

**"But I don't want to have condoms all over the house
where my kids or other people might see them!"**

Of course not. Have them handy, but not necessarily
in plain sight. If you are very concerned about someone
finding them, keep them hidden where you feel they
are safe from discovery until a few hours before you
might use them.

Reassure your partner by saying, *"I know it's difficult
these days and I don't want condoms lying around in view all
over the house either. But I'm sure we can find discreet places
for them, where we can still have them handy."*

**"But AIDS is a gay disease."**

That's a common misunderstanding. The idea that
AIDS is confined to certain groups of people is an
unfortunate byproduct of media sensationalism. It's
what you *do* and *how* you do it that matters—*not* the
kind of person you are.

The fact is this: sexually transmitted diseases, including AIDS, are simply indiscriminate viruses or bacteria,
unable to distinguish between a gay man and a straight
one or between a man and a woman, a rich person and

poor person, a young person and an old person, a married person and a single person, a black person and a white person.

The main factor in AIDS transmission is not sexual preference. The main factor in AIDS transmission is the exchange of body fluids—semen and blood especially. Nearly everyone who is sexually active with others risks AIDS infection; unless you have been in a monogamous relationship for many years (and have avoided all other methods of AIDS infection), you are vulnerable to infection with the AIDS virus.

Tell your partner up front, *"A lot of people used to think that and some still do. But it's simply not true. Anyone can get AIDS, and a lot of people are getting it, not just gay men but straights, too—people like us."*

### *"But I hardly ever have sex."*

The frequency of sex or the number of sexual partners you have had does not necessarily mean you cannot contract a sexually transmitted disease. And with AIDS, a person can be infected with the virus and never know it. Most people who are infected with the AIDS virus do not know, show no symptoms, and are highly infectious to others.

Respond to this by saying, *"Millions of people are infected without knowing it—it may seem unlikely either of us have it, but it is possible. Isn't it better to be safe?"*

**"You don't trust me. I told you I have never been exposed to the AIDS (or herpes) virus."**

Today it is not enough to know that your sexual partner considers himself or herself to be "safe." Regardless of what you or your partner may believe to be the case about past sexual partners, any one former sexual partner may have been infected, and that is enough to have exposed you or your partner to the AIDS virus. With herpes, and with AIDS, it is possible for an individual to be unknowingly infected with the virus and to pass along the infection without any obvious symptoms.

Explain to your partner that you do, indeed, trust him or her, but you have no way of knowing or trusting his or her former partners. Condoms make it safer for both of you.

Again, you should say to your partner, *"It may seem unlikely either of us has been infected but it's possible. I do trust you, but we just don't know for sure."* You might be tempted to agree that your partner doesn't have a disease, but as in the above response, you don't know for certain. Even if your partner doesn't realize it, this response can be a little manipulative. Don't give up on your decision to use a condom because you feel bad that you've seemingly doubted your partner's trust. Say again, *"I'm sorry, but we have no way of knowing right now. I'd feel so much better for both of us if we used condoms—it's not at all that I don't trust you."*

## *"But we've been monogamous for months (or years)."*

This is where we get into tricky timing, because the AIDS virus has been actively infecting people since the late 1970s. Monogamy is no defense against AIDS infection unless neither partner has been infected in the past. If the blood test for antibodies to the AIDS virus is available in your state, it is the surest way to find whether you have been infected. But it can take up to one year from the date of infection for the antibodies to develop, so a blood test would not be absolutely certain unless you were to avoid any possibility of infection from your partner (or from any other source) for one year, and then have your blood tested again.

If you are not going to have the antibody test, then you should use a condom to protect each other from possible infection. And if one partner is infected, you can't assume that because you've been having sex, that the other partner has already been infected. The AIDS virus can be delivered in higher and higher doses each time infected body fluids are exchanged, and scientists don't know just how much of the virus you need to become infected or to become seriously ill.

Say to your partner, *"The experts are still not sure about a lot of things having to do with AIDS. It can take a long time to show up, and lots of people have no symptoms but were infected a long time ago. We just don't know."* Or, if you both have been monogamous for a year or more, you could explain: *"There's a test for the AIDS virus we could both take."*

### *"But condoms don't work."*

This is a common objection, based on the statistic that when used for birth control, condoms have a 10 percent failure rate. Of course, AIDS prevention is not really comparable to birth control, because a person with the AIDS virus is always potentially infectious, but a woman is fertile for only a few days each month.

Because of that 10 percent failure rate, most experts recommend the use of a spermicidal jelly or cream in conjunction with condom use. If you choose a spermicide that contains nonoxynol-9, you are better protected against the AIDS virus if the condom does break in use. Nonoxynol-9 is a substance contained in many spermicides and in many sexual lubricants; it has been shown to kill the AIDS virus on contact.

At the University of California, San Francisco, Dr. Marcus Conant and Dr. Jay Levy conducted a study of condom strength in blocking the AIDS virus. They tested five different condom brands, both latex and natural skin. The doctors filled the condoms with fluid that contained a concentration of AIDS virus 5000 times higher than would be found in semen. The fluid remained in the condoms for up to three weeks without any penetration or leakage of the AIDS virus, even with high pressure applied to the condoms. Dr. Conant believes that if used with a spermicide lubricant containing nonoxynol-9, condoms are safe against AIDS infection during intercourse 100 percent of the time (reported by Michael Helquist, *The Advocate*, August 6, 1985).

Other health experts do not agree, saying that there are no guarantees of 100 percent safety except with abstinence or no-risk sex such as masturbation, hugging, massage, or fantasy. Because the experts do not agree— and because statistics such as these are subject to too many variables and interpretations—we can't say with certainty that even if you use a condom and spermicide, you're safe; we can say you're *safer*. And until a cure or vaccine can be found for AIDS, it's certainly better to be *safer* than sorry.

You can try telling your partner, *"A lot of studies show condoms are very effective in stopping the AIDS virus— especially if we use them with a lubricant called nonoxynol-9."* If your partner still raises this objection, explain: *"Maybe condoms aren't a guarantee, but I think they at least make sex safer for both of us, and I know I'd feel better."*

**"I'm so sick of all this heavy, serious news about disease and condoms."**

If your partner feels that condoms are a reminder of all this serious business, and that this interferes with sex, explain that the most important sexual organ in the body is the mind. It is the mind that keeps sex either lively and fun or serious and grim. There is a place for frolic and humor in safe sexual practices.

One couple we know, to make themselves more comfortable with condoms and to see how strong condoms were, bought a half-dozen different brands and blew each condom up like a giant balloon. They even twisted the inflated condoms into balloon animals and stuck them to the walls with static from their hair and clothes. It may sound ridiculous, but it helped both of them overcome their shyness about condoms.

Despite the serious need for condoms in intercourse, there is no reason why fun can't be a part of your sex life. If your partner misses the good old days before condoms were so necessary, show him or her, with your caring words and actions, that sex can still be plenty of fun.

Reassure your partner by saying, *"I know it's hard—and sometimes it seems like sex can't be fun anymore. But we can get used to condoms. I think really good sex has a lot to do with our thinking and with the mind—we can experiment with condoms as often as you like!"*

### *"I never use those things ... I hate them."*

For a woman, this kind of response might mean that she's always used another form of birth control. A gay man might lack experience using condoms, because it's only been recently that gay couples have discovered a need to use them. And a straight man might respond this way because he's had trouble using condoms in the past—it can be clumsy to use condoms at first—or because he associates condoms only with birth control.

Anyone may have had a partner who hated condoms so much that it became an ordeal to try to use one. And many people simply are unaware of the risks involved in having unprotected sex.

If your partner says that he or she hates condoms and just never uses them, try to find out why. You may have to be very patient, because it's difficult for many people to say what they really feel. If no reasons are offered, ask your partner if he or she will *try* to use condoms with you. Offer to do all the work (buying them, putting them on, getting the right lubricant or spermicide, and so on), and explain as often as necessary why you feel that it is important to use condoms.

Chances are that whatever objection your partner has, you can find the argument and possible response elsewhere in this book. Give your partner a copy of this book, or read it aloud together.

Ask patiently, *"Why do you hate them? Will you try using condoms a few times and see?"* Tell your partner, *"I'll buy them and make sure they're always around. I'll do my best to make it easy to use them—I'd just feel so much better if we used condoms."*

### "Condoms are gross."

This brief statement might seem to be a "case-closed" argument, but try to be patient. Explain all the reasons why condoms are a good idea. Especially tell your lover that you are simply concerned that you may have been exposed to something without knowing, and the last thing you want is for him or her to be exposed also.

Try saying, *"I know you don't like the idea, but condoms are just so important right now. I don't want either of us to* have to take the chance of getting AIDS—there are so many risks and unknowns."

### "Condoms are messy."

Again, this short remark might seem hard to deny. Use calm reasoning. Reassure your lover that with practice and when used correctly, condoms do not have to be messy or awkward. In one way condoms make sex less messy, because the semen is kept contained in the condom.

Tell your partner, "Condoms don't have to be messy—after some practice, I'm sure it won't be any problem. Anyway, some people think it's less messy with a condom since the sperm doesn't get all over the place."

### "I feel as if there's pressure on me to stay erect. Because I can only wear a condom when I'm erect, putting one on and wearing one during sex makes me feel like my 'staying power' is being tested."

Reassure your partner, with words and gestures, that this sort of pressure is the last thing you want him to feel during your lovemaking. Don't wait until you are having sex to discuss this particular point. Bring the subject up ahead of time. Sex is meant to bring pleasure to both partners, but sex doesn't always depend upon whether one partner is erect.

If your partner loses his erection while trying to put on a condom, be understanding. If your partner wants to continue other safe forms of lovemaking without an erection, by all means continue. But if the fact that he is not erect bothers him, don't insist that your lovemaking continue. You want to be especially certain that he doesn't feel any emotional pressure from you on this point, so that future attempts to use a condom aren't problematic.

If he says he feels pressure, reassure him: *"I don't ever want you to feel pressured. But using condoms is something I feel we should do—and I'll do everything I can to help make it easier. It doesn't matter if it's a little awkward at first for both of us. Sex with you is good no matter what."*

### *"Making love with a condom is like taking a shower in a raincoat. It misses the whole point."*

If this is your partner's response, try this explanation: When someone breaks a leg and has to wear a cast, the doctor warns him or her not to get the cast wet. When the person takes showers or bathes he or she wraps the cast in plastic. After the first few times, it is less awkward. By the time the cast comes off, the person is so used to protecting the cast that when taking a shower *without* wrapping the leg in plastic it seems like something is missing.

If people can routinely learn this kind of behavior— when the worst consequence is an extra trip to the doctor —certainly they can learn to cover the penis with a condom to protect their lives.

As to "missing the whole point," sex is much more than inserting the penis until ejaculation. We recommend the new, updated edition of Alex Comfort's book *The Joy of Sex* or John Preston's *Safe Sex* for anyone who does not understand how sex can be much more than intercourse.

Tell your lover, *"I think once we get used to using condoms all the time it will be second nature. And there are all kinds of pleasurable things we can do besides actual intercourse. I just don't feel using condoms will seem that different after a while, especially since it is so crucial to use them."*

**"Condoms make me feel cheap and dirty. Only prostitutes or promiscuous women need to have their partners use them."**

Some women feel this way. It is true that members of the world's oldest profession have been using condoms for a very long time. That's because they *work*. They do prevent pregnancy and the spread of disease. If your partner says that condoms make her feel cheap and dirty, say that this is the last thing you want to make her feel. Tell her that the point of using condoms is to protect both of you, that you care about her health and yours too. Ask her what makes her feel wonderful and what you can do to make her feel good. Be sincere, and when all the talking is finished, remember that actions speak louder than words.

Say to her, *"I know it seems like condoms carry a kind of*

*'reputation,' but that's because they've worked for hundreds of years to prevent disease or pregnancy. I don't ever want you to feel that using condoms makes you cheap or dirty. I simply care a great deal about your health. Whatever makes you feel happy and excited, let me know—I'll do my best to make you feel good."*

## "But we don't need to use condoms. We already use effective birth control."

Even if you are using effective birth control, it is wise to use condoms during sex. Sexually transmitted diseases such as AIDS, herpes, gonorrhea, and syphilis cannot be stopped by birth control pills, diaphragms, IUDs, or spermicides. Although there is evidence that spermicides that contain nonoxynol-9 can lessen the risk of infection by the AIDS virus, only the condom used properly has been shown to prevent the transmission of the AIDS virus during intercourse. So tell your partner that only the use of a condom will protect you both from the spread of sexually transmitted disease.

You could say, *"I know we don't have to worry about birth control, but with AIDS and so many other diseases around, we need to do what we can to be safer when we have sex. There's so much we don't know yet, especially about AIDS, but we do know that using condoms is one good way of protecting us."*

### For any other argument that sounds defensive:

Defensiveness, which can arise from fear, confusion, or frustration, may be expressed in many different ways. If you meet with a reaction that sounds like a refusal to face facts, you need to be gentle and sympathetic. If your partner doesn't know the facts about disease, tell him or her. If your partner is afraid, be reassuring. Tell him or her that yes, things *are* scary, but there is something you can do about it.

Remember, the spread of AIDS is a crisis, not just another nuisance of modern life. Disagreeable reactions, depression, and even temporary loss of sexual desire are common and understandable. And to avoid these bad feelings, people may pretend that the problem doesn't apply to them. Be patient and be caring. You have everything to gain from persuading your lover to use a condom.

## A SPECIAL PLEA TO WOMEN

### *"If I don't do as he says he'll leave me."*

If you find yourself thinking this way, it's time to reconsider your situation. Acting on the fear that a man will leave you if you don't cater to his every wish could be deadly when it comes to not using condoms. Some men use intimidation to get their way, and to the women who love them—or who fear losing them—it works. Here are some of the ways a man might use your fear of losing him or take advantage of your insecurity:

*"How can you deny me my greatest pleasure?"*

*"Who are you to tell me what I should and shouldn't do? I've been having sex for years, and I've never used condoms."*

*"If you loved me you would do as I ask;"* or *"But I thought you loved me;"* or *"I guess you don't feel as strongly about me as you say you do."*

These last lines have been used for years to talk a woman into having sex. But when they are used to talk a woman out of using condoms, they show not just selfishness on the man's part, but a dangerous disregard for life.

Not giving in to a man you love is worth the risk of losing him when the stakes are this high. It is self-destructive to continue in a relationship with someone who risks your life every time you make love. In addition to the real risk of contracting AIDS from a man who most likely would not know if he were infected, the stress of uncertainty would intrude into your sex life and undoubtedly affect the relationship.

To counter such a line, any of the following phrases can be used to start a discussion:

*"Let's talk about this 'love' you want me to prove. Do you really want to be 'loved' by having someone risk her life for you? I'd much rather show my love by protecting you and myself."*

*"Don't you see that by using condoms we're both showing our love for each other? If any former partner of yours was infected with this thing, she could have infected you. Neither of you would know it, but, in fact, you could be infecting me every time we make love. I could be infecting you unknowingly, too."*

*"I can think of lots of ways I show my love for you that are not dangerous. I listen to you/cook for you/ surprise you with gifts or notes/I'm your ally/friend/best buddy/loyal companion. I think of you/call you/make love to you/hug you. What I want in return takes less time than any of these things, and shows me that you respect me and value the love I show you day in and day out."*

*"I understand that you're not sure of my love. But if I were to demonstrate my love by not using condoms, how would you be sure of my love when we were not having sex?"*

*"I really wish I could ignore the whole issue of condoms, but the way things are these days, I can't. If you insist that we don't use them, I will insist that we practice safe sex only, and that we avoid intercourse completely. I know I can satisfy you in other ways."*

*"I do love you, but I refuse to demonstrate my love with such a tremendous risk. I suppose you will just have to doubt my love, or find someone who loves you more than she loves her own life."*

It may be very difficult for you to stand up to a man with such an assertive point of view, but it is urgent that you do. It is very likely that the man does not understand the nature of the AIDS virus. You can explain to him that even you might be infected, and that you are protecting him, too, by asking him to use condoms.

Denying someone you love something he wants can be hard. But it is an effort worth pursuing, because you are worth it!

## A WORD ABOUT MONOGAMY

Even when two people are in a monogamous relationship, neither partner can be 100 percent certain that the other is faithful. Some people are emotionally loyal to their partners and don't consider an occasional physical dalliance to count as an "extramarital affair." To some people even one fling would not change their self image, and they would still think of themselves as monogamous. Yet that occasional affair or that single fling could have infected the straying partner.

It is important that you and your partner communicate honestly about the nature and degree of fidelity you want from one another. If your relationship has been based on a "What I don't know won't hurt me" understanding, that premise is no longer true. If either of you has been unfaithful in the last ten years, you should use a condom for intercourse until a blood test (twelve months after having safe sex only) confirms that you are not infected with the AIDS virus.

For centuries, straying partners who have been infected with sexually transmitted diseases have had to protect their spouses. Introducing protection where there was never the need before can be a test of the relationship, and can be the most difficult thing you'll ever have to do. But for the sake of your health and your future, it is worth doing. Only you know if you are at risk from having had sex with someone else. Only you can protect your partner from the consequences of that risk.

If you have risked infection, you should not have unprotected sex until you have a blood test for the AIDS virus (a year after the last time you had unprotected sex). Use condoms with your partner or practice only safe sex that does not require a condom (see below). This could be the time to introduce some creative lovemaking into the relationship. Avoiding unprotected intercourse could lead to new ways of expressing your love and new ways of giving your partner pleasure.

Finally, if you're ever going to have sex outside your relationship, use condoms every time.

## SAFE SEX AND OTHER CONSIDERATIONS

These are frightening times. Daily news stories create worry and anxiety. This tension takes its toll in our lives and in our relationships. That is why it is especially important to communicate openly with your lover about the need for condoms.

If you can express your sexual desires and talk with your partner about ways to satisfy those desires safely, then you can reduce your own stress level and help maintain good health.

Some of you may never enjoy using condoms. There are an infinite number of ways to make love without having intercourse. Good sex is sex that satisfies both partners, physically and emotionally.

So if you can't persuade your lover to use a condom, *make love safely anyway by practicing other forms of safe sex.*

Just what is safe sex? "Safe sex" is sex without risk of infection, sex that does not involve the exchange of body fluids. It is sex that is protected with condoms or sex that does not require condoms to be safe, such as massage, mutual masturbation, dry kissing (no tongues), caressing, and fantasy.

Many public health departments have created a list of sexual activities that are considered safe, possibly safe, and unsafe. "Safe" means that you cannot contract AIDS (or most sexually transmitted diseases) by doing these things. "Possibly safe" means that the experts aren't completely sure about the risks of infection by AIDS or other STDs if you do these things. But with care and good hygiene, they are possibly safe. "Unsafe" means just that—these practices can lead to infection with the AIDS virus as well as other STDs.

The San Francisco Bay Area Physicians for Human Rights classifies sexual activities as follows:

## SAFE

Massage, hugging
Mutual masturbation
Social kissing (dry)
Body-to-body rubbing
Fantasy, voyeurism, exhibitionism

## POSSIBLY SAFE

French kissing (wet)
Anal intercourse with condom
Vaginal intercourse with condom
Fellatio (oral sex on a man)—stop
    before climax
Cunnilingus (oral sex on a woman)
Watersports (sexual activity involving
    urine)—external only

## UNSAFE

Rimming (oral–anal contact)
Fisting
Blood contact
Sharing sex toys or needles
Semen or urine in mouth
Anal intercourse without condom
Vaginal intercourse without condom

## ONE FINAL THOUGHT . . .

If you can't persuade your partner to use a condom, then you'll want to persuade him or her to engage in safe sexual practices only. But if your partner won't use a condom or practice safe sex, you'll want to consider not having sex at all with that person. If you're in a relationship, you can take some time to discuss it and think it over. If you've just met the person, it's especially important that you bring up the subject before you get into a sexual situation. Remember that you are in charge of your body and your life. If a partner attempts to coerce you into any sexual activity, you can leave, call for help, or fight back.

# PART THREE

# ... AND WHY YOU SHOULD

Intimacy these days is a call to responsibility. This is a crisis time. It's normal and okay to feel confused, irritated, even angry—as though the rug has been pulled out from under you. Three factors are forcing us to reexamine our sex lives: (1) the spread of sexually transmitted diseases, especially AIDS; (2) the high rate of unwanted pregnancies; and (3) the decreasing safety reassurances of other forms of birth control.

Though this is a crisis time, it doesn't have to be devastating, and we can approach these issues realistically. Becoming more informed—learning what we can do—can help reduce our confusion and anger. This section presents the facts about sexually transmitted diseases and birth control.

## SEXUALLY TRANSMITTED DISEASES AND CONDOMS

*AIDS.*   Acquired immune deficiency syndrome (AIDS) is a disease that breaks down the body's natural ability to fight infection. This, in time, leads to death, and there is no known cure.

AIDS is caused by a virus that can be transmitted during sex. The virus is the human immunodeficiency virus (HIV). This virus is present in the blood and semen of infected individuals. Not everyone who is infected with the AIDS virus comes down with the full-blown disease. Infected individuals may remain free from symptoms or illness, and thus may not even know that they have been infected. Individuals who are unaware of their infection may pass the virus on to others without suspecting it. Tests that detect your exposure to the AIDS virus are available in some states. Ask your doctor for more information, or call your public health department, sex information line, or crisis hotline.

The AIDS virus is transmitted through the exchange of certain body fluids. This means you must avoid coming into contact with infected blood or semen, during sex and at other times as well. Because you cannot know who is infected (without a blood test and absolute trust that your partner has been monogamous since that blood test), to reduce your risk of infection you should avoid contact with any blood or semen, at all times, including menstrual blood.

Condoms are effective in preventing the transmission of the AIDS virus because they provide a barrier between body fluids that may be infected with the AIDS virus and body tissues that might absorb the virus. Semen and blood can contain the AIDS virus, and the walls of the vagina, mouth, and rectum may be receptive to the virus.

Using condoms every time you have sex can greatly

reduce the risk of being infected with the AIDS virus. If you are already infected with the AIDS virus, using condoms can reduce the risk of your being reinfected with even higher doses of the virus and can help prevent you from spreading the virus to others.

*GONORRHEA.*  Gonorrhea is a bacterial infection of the sexual organs. You get it by having sexual contact with someone who is infected, and it takes from one to ten days for the infection to take hold once you've been exposed. It can be cured with antibiotics.

Condoms are highly effective in preventing infection from gonorrhea, because they do not allow the bacteria to come into contact with either the penis or the vagina.

*SYPHILIS.*  Syphilis is a bacterial infection of the sexual organs. You get it by having sexual contact with someone who has it or by coming into contact with a syphilis sore (chancre). It takes from ten to ninety days after contact for signs of infection to appear. Syphilis can be cured with antibiotics.

Condoms can prevent syphilis to a high degree, because they do not allow the syphilis bacteria to come into contact with either the penis or vagina. Syphilis sores may, however, occur on the mouth or other parts of the body that are unprotected by a condom.

*HERPES.*  Herpes is an infection caused by a virus. You get it by having sexual contact with someone who has it or by coming into contact with a herpes sore. You can get it from someone who has it even if that person is not having an outbreak of herpes sores. (Spreading herpes this way is called shedding the virus.) It takes from two to twenty days after contact for signs of infection to appear, and there is no cure. Herpes sores can be treated with medication, but the underlying viral infection is not curable.

Condoms are highly effective in preventing the spread of the herpes virus during intercourse; however, herpes can also be transmitted through kissing.

*NON-GONOCOCCAL URETHRITIS and INFECTIONS.* These used to be called NSU (for non-specific urethritis) or other nonspecific infections of the vagina, but we have since learned that the most common cause of such infections is an organism called chlamydia. You get it by having sexual contact with someone who has it, and the amount of time from infection until you come down with symptoms varies widely. Chlamydia can cause sterility in women. Antibiotics can be prescribed to treat and cure these infections.

Condoms are very effective in preventing transmission of these infections, because they provide a barrier between the infected individual and his or her partner.

*VENEREAL WARTS.* Venereal warts are caused by a virus that causes painless or slightly itching small bumps that grow around the sex organs, anus, or mouth. You get them from sexual contact with someone who has them, and it takes from one to six months for them to show up after infection. They can be treated and cured with a variety of techniques by a doctor.

Condoms can be of some use in preventing the transmission of venereal warts, because—depending on the location of the warts—the condom could provide a barrier between the infected area and the other partner.

*HTLV-I.*   Although very little is known, there are some early reports that infection from a virus called human T-cell leukemia virus (HTLV-I) may be responsible for a rare and virulent form of leukemia or a severe nerve disease known as tropical spastic paraparesis (TSP). Researchers suspect that the virus is spread in the same way as the AIDS virus—through unprotected sexual contact, blood contact, or sharing of syringes.

Although research is only beginning, we presume that condoms could help in reducing the risk of sexually transmitted infection by HTLV-I.

## BIRTH CONTROL: THE FACTS TODAY

Today there is increasing concern about contraceptives. New research and awareness have made many people leery of the intrauterine device (IUD) and the pill because of their medical side effects. The sponge and the diaphragm can also cause problems, and some women find them awkward to use. For those who feel that these birth control methods are unsatisfactory, the condom remains a safe, practical alternative.

The facts on different kinds of contraceptives follow, so that you can judge for yourself the pros and cons of each method.

## CONDOM

### How Does It Work?
The condom is a protective rubber covering that fits

on the penis. It might also be made from a natural membrane. The condom keeps the man's semen from entering the vagina.

### How Effective Is It?
The condom is very effective in preventing pregnancy when used correctly and used every time the couple has sex. When the condom is used alone, it is 90 percent to 98 percent effective. If it is used along with a spermicide the effectiveness is 98+ percent.

### Benefits and Advantages
1. There are no health risks or medical side effects to either partner.
2. You need to use it only during sex (unlike the Pill, for example).
3. They are easy to buy and to have handy.
4. They are very effective.
5. You do not need to have a prescription or a medical exam.
6. They are inexpensive.
7. They may protect against cervical cancer.

### Problems and Disadvantages
1. They can be used incorrectly and thus ineffectively.
2. On rare occasions a man or woman might be allergic to the rubber. Changing to a natural membrane condom can solve this problem.
3. Occasionally, the man reports a blunting of sexual sensation.

### Other Comments and Information
Condoms can be bought in many places, including

drugstores, clinics, adult bookstores, and some large supermarkets. They can also be found in vending machines, although there is the possibility that these condoms will be old and therefore not as good. It is an excellent idea to use a spermicide with the condom to increase its effectiveness. Spermicide can be purchased in most of the same places where condoms are purchased.

## THE PILL

### How Does It Work?
The Pill contains hormones that keep the ovaries from releasing eggs. Pregnancy cannot occur when there is no egg to fertilize (no ovulation).

### How Effective Is It?
The Pill is highly effective. When the Pill is used correctly (it must be taken every day), the effectiveness rate is 98 percent to 99 percent.

### Benefits and Advantages
1. The Pill is very effective.
2. The woman's period is often more regular and cramps are often less painful.
3. It is easy to use and does not interrupt sex.
4. It may lower the chances of getting ovarian cysts, cancer of the ovaries and uterus, and anemia.

### Problems and Disadvantages
1. It does not prevent the spread of sexually transmitted disease.

2. There can be side effects, especially during the first months of usage, which include nausea, retention of fluid, missed periods, spotting between periods, vaginal infections, weight gain, and changes in mood.
3. Major medical problems can occur, but rarely. These include blood clots, an increase in the chance of heart attack (especially if the user smokes), and, only very rarely, liver tumors. There is also a slightly higher chance of getting gallbladder disease, and some women who take the Pill get high blood pressure.
4. Other side effects include facial skin discoloration, which can be permanent, and some women have trouble getting pregnant for a short while after stopping the Pill.
5. A medical exam and a prescription are required.
6. The Pill must be taken on a regular daily schedule.

### Other Comments and Information

Both estrogen and progesterone, the female hormones, are contained in the Pill. (There is also a mini-pill, which contains only progesterone.) There are sometimes medical reasons why a woman cannot take the Pill. If you miss a day or two, use a backup method. If you forget for three days, call your doctor.

## THE INTRAUTERINE DEVICE (IUD)

### How Does It Work?

The IUD is a small device inserted by a doctor into the uterus. No one really knows how it works. Experts think the IUD creates a hostile environment for the egg, thus keeping it from attaching itself to the lining of the uterus.

### How Effective Is It?
The effectiveness is about 95 percent.

### Benefits and Advantages
1. When it stays in place, it is usually effective for a year, and is there whenever it is needed.
2. When properly placed, it is usually not felt by either the man or the woman.

### Problems and Disadvantages
1. It provides no protection from sexually transmitted diseases.
2. The IUD is available only by prescription and must be inserted by a clinician or doctor.
3. The placement must be checked after each period.
4. Bleeding and increased cramping might occur.
5. It can slip out of position.
6. The uterus can become infected or punctured.
7. If you become pregnant, there can be difficulties (increased chances of tubal pregnancy, for example).
8. Chances of pelvic inflammatory disease are increased.

### Other Comments and Information
If you experience unusual discharge or cramping, heavy bleeding, fever or chills, call the doctor immediately.

## DIAPHRAGM

### How Does It Work?

The diaphragm is a piece of rubber with a flexible rim that fits snugly in the vagina over the cervix. It prevents the sperm from entering the opening to the uterus. The spermicide, which must be used with the diaphragm, destroys any sperm that might reach the uterus.

### How Effective Is It?

The effectiveness is estimated to be 80 percent to 98 percent, depending on how carefully it is used.

### Benefits and Advantages

1. The diaphragm can be put in place a couple of hours before sex.
2. There are no major medical side effects.

### Problems and Disadvantages

1. It offers no protection from sexually transmitted diseases.
2. A medical exam is required for the fitting of the diaphragm, and it can be purchased only with a prescription.
3. There is an increased chance of getting a urinary tract infection.
4. On rare occasions, a man or a woman might be allergic to either the rubber or the spermicide.

### Other Comments and Information

The diaphragm must be used with a spermicide.

# VAGINAL SPONGE

### How Does It Work?

The sponge contains a spermicide, and after it is moistened with water it is inserted into the vagina. Once in place, it both blocks and destroys the sperm.

### How Effective Is It?

Because it has not been studied for long, it is difficult to give an accurate estimate, but some experts put the effectiveness rate at 85 percent to 90 percent.

### Benefits and Advantages

1. The sponge is effective for twenty-four hours once it is inserted into the vagina. This means you can insert it up to twenty-four hours before having sex, or you can have sex—as often as you want—within the twenty-four hours following insertion. (Unlike the diaphragm, it does not have to be changed after each use within the twenty-four hour period.) You do have to leave the sponge in place for at least six to eight hours after intercourse.
2. It can be bought without a prescription.

### Problems and Disadvantages

1. It provides no protection from sexually transmitted diseases.
2. The sponge is relatively new—side effects or problems have yet to be discovered.
3. It may be hard to remove, and might break into pieces.
4. It can be expensive.
5. On rare occasions, a man or woman might be allergic

to the chemicals contained in the sponge.
6. It can irritate the lining of the vagina.
7. For women who have given birth, the sponge is not as effective.
8. Researchers believe the sponge may cause toxic shock syndrome, but only very rarely.

### Other Comments and Information
The sponge must be left in place for several hours following sex.

# VAGINAL SPERMICIDE

### How Does It Work?
Various forms of spermicides (jellies, creams, suppositories, and foam) are inserted into the vagina. The sperm are destroyed when they come into contact with the spermicide.

### How Effective Is It?
When used by itself, it is estimated to be 70 percent to 90 percent effective. (The wide range reflects its unpredictability.) If used with a condom, the effectiveness is estimated at 98+ percent.

### Benefits and Advantages
1. There are no major medical side effects.
2. It can be bought without a prescription at various stores.

### Problems and Disadvantages

1. It provides no protection from sexually transmitted diseases. Spermicides containing nonoxynol-9 provide some protection from the AIDS virus, but doctors do not believe that, by itself, nonoxynol-9 offers *adequate* protection against AIDS.
2. It must be inserted in the vagina very shortly before intercourse (about twenty minutes to one hour).
3. Spermicide used alone can be messy.
4. Used alone, it is not one of the highly effective methods.

### Other Comments and Information

Spermicide is best used along with a condom or diaphragm.

## RHYTHM METHOD OR FERTILITY AWARENESS METHOD

### How Does It Work?

The woman can learn to tell the time when she can get pregnant and not have sex during those times.

### How Effective Is It?

Like the use of spermicide alone, this method is unpredictable in its effectiveness. Estimates of effectiveness range from 76 percent to 98 percent.

### Benefits and Advantages

1. There are no major medical side effects.
2. This method is very inexpensive; only a vaginal thermometer and a rectal thermometer need be purchased.

### Problems and Disadvantages

1. It provides no protection from sexually transmitted diseases.
2. The woman should take a class to learn the method.
3. Vaginal and rectal temperatures must be checked each day.
4. When it is an unsafe time, another method must be used or the couple should not have sex.

### Other Comments and Information

If this method is used, it requires very careful attention. The low end of the effectiveness rate indicates a potentially high failure rate.

## PERMANENT METHODS

### How Does It Work?

*Tubal ligation:* A surgical procedure in which the woman's fallopian tubes are blocked. Once done, the egg is prevented from reaching a point where sperm can fertilize it.

*Vasectomy:* A surgical procedure in which the man's vas deferens (tubes that carry the sperm) are cut and tied. Once this operation has been performed, the ejaculate, which is still released at climax, contains no sperm.

### How Effective Is It?

Both methods are 99+ percent effective.

### Benefits and Advantages

1. It is the most effective method of birth control.
2. There is no need to follow a regular regime or to worry about birth control each time you have sex.

### Problems and Disadvantages

1. It provides no protection from sexually transmitted diseases.
2. There is no changing one's mind; both methods are almost always irreversible.
3. You must have an operation, and there is some pain shortly afterward.
4. There is a small chance of a minor infection following surgery.
5. Following checkups are necessary to see if the vas deferens has grown back.

### Other Comments and Information

This method is obviously one that requires a great deal of careful consideration beforehand.

# PART FOUR
# ALL ABOUT CONDOMS

## QUESTIONS AND ANSWERS

Many people hesitate to use condoms simply because they don't know much about them. In this section we raise some common questions about condoms and provide answers to those questions.

**Q** *Where do you buy condoms? And how are they packaged?*

**A** You can buy condoms at pharmacies, some clinics, adult bookstores, large supermarkets, and vending machines in public restrooms. Nowadays condoms are also sold at gift stores in gay neighborhoods in large cities. Condoms are given away free at some places, such as health clinics, doctors' offices, retail stores featuring sexual materials, and gay bars.

Condoms are individually packaged in cellophane or foil wrappers. Sometimes they are available singly, but most often they are available in small boxes of three, six, or a dozen. Some pharmacies keep condoms behind the counter, and others display them alongside appropriate lubricants. Don't hesitate to ask the pharmacist to help you. He or she is a professional and can answer your questions.

**Q** *Which are better—latex condoms or natural condoms?*

**A** Natural-membrane condoms are made from sheep's gut. Some men find that a natural condom's texture, wetness, and slickness feel really good. Latex condoms are manufactured from synthetic materials. Both kinds are strong, durable, and prevent disease and pregnancy. The only problem with natural membrane condoms is that the density of the natural membrane can be unequal. That means that the wall of the condom may not be uniformly thick and might leak more easily than a condom made of latex.

**Q** *Do condoms come in different sizes? What if it feels too tight? What if it feels too large or baggy?*

**A** In the United States, one size fits all. The latex from which most condoms are made is extremely elastic, and can stretch to fit any size. The same is true of natural membrane condoms. In fact, in product testing, condoms are stretched and inflated to several times their original size and shape in order to test their strengths and limits. They are put under much more stress than a condom would usually receive during sexual intercourse.

A major complaint that some men have about fit is that condoms often seem too short—when completely unrolled, they do not reach all the way to the base of the penis. When this is the case they restrict full movement during intercourse because the friction of intercourse rolls the condom up off the penis. This problem of unrolling during intercourse brings an undue amount of attention to the condom. Some men even hold it in place with their hand.

One solution is to use the brands of condoms that include a light adhesive at the base, which helps the condom remain in place.

**Q** *But doesn't the condom need to fit all the way to the base of the penis?*

**A** For ease of movement during intercourse, that would be ideal. But for protection, it isn't necessary. The two major barriers of protection a condom provides are to trap the semen at ejaculation and to prevent skin-to-skin (that is, mucous membrane-to-mucous membrane) contact during intercourse. The shaft of the penis is covered with normal skin. It is the canal of the penis that is mucous membrane and is in need of a barrier for protection for both partners against AIDS, gonorrhea, and chlamydia. In addition, normal skin can have a herpes or syphilis sore. If a condom covers this infected skin, it affords significant protection against transmitting herpes or syphilis.

**Q** *What about different shaped condoms? What is a receptacle tip?*

**A** Many brands of condoms have a little built-in tapered space at the very top. The purpose of this receptacle tip (sometimes called a reservoir) is to catch the semen when it is ejaculated. Condoms with or without receptacle tips are effective barriers.

When you use condoms that don't have a reservoir, leave a small space at the tip of the condom so that there is room to catch the semen.

It's okay if you forget to leave room or do not have a receptacle tip condom. They are meant only to increase your comfort during ejaculation.

**Q** *What about condoms that are lubricated? What does that mean? Is it necessary?*

**A** Lubrication is not necessary, but many people like the feel of lubricated condoms because they are moist and slippery. Because the condom is rolled, the lubricant is on the outside and inside of a condom. The lubricant can be either gel or silicone, and some lubricants include nonoxynol-9, the spermicide which may help kill the AIDS virus as well as sperm if the condom breaks or slips off. Even if a condom is already lubricated with a spermicide, you can still use more spermicidal jelly. It never hurts to use spermicidal jelly in addition to condoms.

**Q** *If the condom is lubricated, will we need still more* *lubricant? And if the condom is the dry kind, do we need lubrication for that?*

**A**  In either case, additional lubrication may be necessary for comfort during intercourse. The important thing is that you must use a water-based lubricant (such as KY jelly) with condoms. Lubricants that are oil-based (such as petroleum jelly) will cause the latex of the condom to deteriorate, which may lead to breakage. Water-based lubricants will not affect the quality of the latex or natural membrane fibers. You can tell whether the lubricant is water based or oil based by reading the ingredients. Vegetable-based lubricants are oil-based.

**Q**  *Are thicker condoms stronger?*

**A**  Not necessarily. Condom manufacturers produce a number of different brands. Some are thinner than others. All of them work. The purpose of thinner condoms is to provide more sensation for the penis.

**Q**  *Some condoms are available in different colors. Does this make any difference?*

**A**  Colors don't matter for disease prevention or birth control. They may provide you with more visual stimulation, making condoms more fun. But there are no guarantees about the stability of the dyes used to color them. This means that once they are wet, the color may run, which could be startling (but not harmful). The colors may stain sheets or clothing, but will not affect safety.

**Q** *Do condoms ever slip off inside your partner during intercourse?*

**A** Rarely. This is why it's important, though, to use a spermicide or lubricant containing nonoxynol-9. Using an adhesive condom, which has a light adhesive to help it cling to the penis, will help prevent the condom from slipping off. In case this ever does happen, just reach up with your fingers and remove the condom.

The condom is more likely to slip off if the man waits until he is losing his erection before he withdraws his penis from his partner. Either partner can hold onto the condom as the man wearing it withdraws.

**Q** *What about ribbed condoms?*

**A** Ribbed condoms have little ridges on the outside that provide added sensation for the receptive partner during intercourse. Some people find them pleasurable; others find them irritating.

Some condoms are also made with ticklers. These are little ridges or fingerlike attachments at the tip that are designed to create added sensation for the receptive partner. In Japan, the use of fancy condoms is widespread. Some Japanese brands even include floral designs. In the United States plainer brands are the most popular. With the growing popularity of condoms, though, this may change.

**Q** *What about the taste and smell of condoms? Is there anything to be careful about? Is it okay to put them in your mouth?*

**A** Different brands have different tastes and smells. We don't know of any dangers involved in putting latex condoms in your mouth—for oral sex, for example. Some latex condoms have a distinct rubbery smell. Some are absolutely neutral. Some condoms are perfumed and some are dusted with powder. If you are sensitive to such allergens, you might want to be careful with scented or powdered condoms. Try different brands to find the one that suits you. Natural-membrane condoms, however, shouldn't be put in your mouth because of the preservative used in packaging. See the answer about oral sex on page 77.

**Q** *How long do condoms keep? When do they expire?*

**A** This is an important question. If properly stored in a cool place, condoms should last about five years. But they will deteriorate very fast if exposed to heat or sunlight, or if they receive rough treatment. This means that if you are storing condoms in your car's glove compartment or if you are carrying them around in your wallet or purse, you should not leave them there for several months at a time before you use them. When in doubt about a condom's age or condition, throw it out and use a newer one.

**Q** *Are some condoms considered cool and other considered uncool?*

**A** Some major brands of condoms have names that have become synonymous with the word *condom*, and they carry all the clout that comes with that kind of product identification. But other brands are popular among different groups of people. It's really a matter of individual taste.

**Q** *Do condoms vary in quality? What are the good brands? Are there any bad brands to watch out for?*

**A** Although we cannot evaluate the quality or recommend specific brands of condoms, they do vary in quality. As with many other products, people have often used price as an index to quality. But with the introduction of imported condoms and new manufacturers springing up with competitive pricing, to use price as the only indicator of quality might be shortsighted.

The best thing is to talk to people about the brands they know about. A druggist at a pharmacy should be able to answer your questions. It might seem embarrassing to discuss this with a pharmacist, but remember, a pharmacist is like a doctor—with a dedication to service and a clinical approach. Other individuals may be able to advise you as well—talk to your doctor, father, mother, or trusted friends. Many people today have experience with condoms, and many more are just learning about condoms. So there are many folks who are trying to learn and are willing—and need—to talk about condoms.

As for comfort and fit, it's always all right to experiment. Try different brands. See what feels comfortable. Find what you like best.

**Q** *Experiment? Couldn't that be risky? What if a poor brand broke?*

**A** You don't have to experiment with condoms *during* intercourse or even with your partner present. In fact, if you're new to condoms or are trying to find the comfortable brand, it's wise to experiment with them outside of intercourse.

Masturbating with condoms is a good way to become familiar with them in a no-risk, low-pressure setting. You can masturbate alone or with a partner, and you might want to try this many times until you're comfortable and confident using condoms.

Experimentation can take the form of erotic play— alone or with your partner. You can take them out of their packets, unroll them, inspect them, test their elasticity and strength, observe their color, texture, and sensitivity. You can try them on and practice, to see which brand provides the best sensitivity and the most comfortable fit.

Or you can take a clinical approach, simply laying them out on the table some afternoon, inspecting and comparing different brands.

To allay fears about strength and durability, one method of experimentation is to slip your hand into the condom. Once the condom is on your hand, stretch your fingers, clench your fist. This will give you an idea of their strength and flexibility, as well as provide a method of discovering how sensitive the condom is for touch.

Fingernails tear condoms easily. If your condom tears while you are examining it with your hands, remember that with normal, careful use during sex, that most likely won't happen. You'll probably be surprised at how sturdy they are.

**Q** *How do you put a condom on? How careful do you have to be?*

**A** You open the foil or cellophane packet by tearing off any edge. It is like opening a package of ketchup. There is sometimes a small notch that shows where to rip the packet open. Take the condom out of its wrapper. A condom has an inside and an outside. When you place the rounded top of the unrolled condom onto the head of the penis, the rolls of the condom should be facing out, away from the penis, so that you can just unroll it down the length of the penis without much pressure or tugging. It sounds more complicated than it is. And it doesn't really matter if you unroll it inside out—except that if you put it inside out, you might have to tug at it too much and risk tearing it.

You should be careful, of course, because you don't want it to tear. Ripping the condom when tearing open the foil packet is one of the most common causes of breakage. You can avoid this by gently shaking the condom down in the packet before tearing it open. Condoms are fairly strong, but if you snap them or catch them on a fingernail, they can tear. So you do want to be careful, but there's no need to be fearful.

**Q** *Should the penis be completely erect before putting it on?*

**A** Not necessarily. But it is easiest to unroll a condom on a fully or partially erect penis. It is difficult to unroll a condom on a soft penis, and trying to do that can tear the condom. Because the condom is intended to protect both partners during intercourse and possibly during oral sex, you may want to put on the condom before a full erection is reached.

**Q** *Is it any different putting a condom on an uncircumcised penis?*

**A** The procedure for putting on and wearing a condom is the same for uncircumcised men. When the penis is erect, the foreskin is pulled back and the shaft and head of the penis form an uninterrupted line. So putting the condom on is the same. During intercourse the movement of the foreskin usually does not affect the condom. Occasionally the motion will cause the condom to roll up or roll off, but this is unlikely. You can use your hand or your partner's hand to hold the condom in place, or a small piece of masking tape or surgical tape at the base of the condom will solve the problem. Also, some condoms have adhesive at the base. Some men find that wearing the condom inside out keeps the condom from rolling up. (If you are going to try wearing the condom inside out, be very careful unrolling it onto your penis! Don't let a fingernail tear the condom. And be especially careful if you are partially unrolling it before you put it on.)

**Q** *Do women ever put condoms on their partners?*

**A** Yes, many women take an active role, making condom use itself a part of foreplay. Putting a condom on need not be difficult or embarrassing. The manner in which a condom is placed on a penis can be stimulating for the male. In fact, some men feel so much pressure about finding the right moment to put the condom on, that they fear loss of erection. In that case, placing a condom on an erect penis in a sensuous manner could help allay such fears.

**Q** *Do condoms break often? How reliable are they?*

**A** Condoms do not break often. Condom manufacturers have to meet federal standards in their production. And condom manufacturers conduct regular tests on the strength, durability, and reliability of the condoms they manufacture.

If you're especially worried about breakage, you and your partner should develop more confidence in condom use. Try masturbating with condoms until you are comfortable and confident about them. This confidence will result from your experience. And your experience will have been gained without risk.

As long as you are using condoms properly, and are using the right lubricant (water-based, as discussed on page 67), condoms are very reliable. Also see the discussion about condom safety in Part Two, page 27.

**Q** *Do condoms need to be changed?*

**A** Yes. Use a new condom every time you have sex.

Many people, though, enjoy a variety of activities that do not always lead directly to climax. Some people enjoy penetration for a while, then proceed to do other things before returning to another insertion. Periods between penetration are ideal times to change to a new condom if you want to. It is not, however, necessary.

If you and your partner practice a variety of activities, a fresh condom should be used for each one. *A condom used during vaginal intercourse should be replaced before anal intercourse, and vice versa.* The bacteria that normally reside in the vagina and in the anus can lead to infection if transferred from one place to the other.

**Q** *Is there anything special to know about taking the condom off?*

**A** You just pull it off. After intercourse and ejaculation, the condom will be quite wet and slippery, so it will just slide off. Most men use a towel to wipe the ejaculate and lubricant from the penis after removing the condom.

**Q** *What if some of the semen touches me after the condom is off? Can a woman get pregnant? Can I catch any disease from sleeping on a wet spot or if the condom spills semen on me when we're taking it off?*

**A** No, women cannot get pregnant from having semen spilled onto the outside of their bodies. It would be highly unlikely, but if semen should come into contact with any part of the vagina—even the outer lips—it is possible to become pregnant. But we stress that this is a long shot. Neither can you catch a sexually transmitted disease by coming into contact with ejaculate on the outside of the body.

You do not have to worry about pregnancy or sexually transmitted disease from sleeping on a wet spot or having semen spill onto your skin. Sexually transmitted diseases are usually spread by getting a virus or bacteria onto receptive mucous membrane. Regular skin is not mucous membrane. Regular skin resists infection, unless it is broken by cuts or scratches.

**Q** *How do you discard a condom?*

**A** You can simply throw it away. Many people wrap them in tissue or toilet paper first, to be sure they don't spill on the floor. Condoms should not be flushed down the toilet, because they can clog the plumbing.

**Q** *Is oral sex safe? Do we need a condom for oral sex?*

**A**   No one is sure. Doctors and health experts say that fellatio (oral sex performed on a man) without a condom is "possibly safe." They also say that cunnilingus (oral sex performed on a woman) is "possibly safe." That means that they aren't sure just how safe it is. Many people are using condoms for fellatio. This protects against AIDS transmission as well as the spread of gonorrhea, syphilis, and venereal warts. If you use a condom for oral sex, it is best to use an unlubricated brand and to wipe off the latex dust with a towel beforehand.

In order to make oral sex with condoms more palatable, many couples are using flavored lubricants. Available at some pharmacies, sex shops, and adult bookstores, flavored lubricants are an option you might want to consider using if you find the rubber taste of latex condoms unpleasant.

If you're going to use a condom for oral sex, use only the latex brand. Natural membrane condoms are packaged with a small bit of formaldehyde as a preservative. There is probably not enough formaldehyde to cause any real harm, but it is something that should not be put in the mouth.

As for cunnilingus, precautions could include using an oral or dental dam. A dental dam is a piece of latex that dentists use in various procedures. It's just a small square of latex very much like the material that condoms are made of. Safe sex practitioners have adapted dental dams for protection in oral sex—by placing a dental dam over the vaginal or anal opening, a barrier is provided that protects the tongue from direct contact. But dental dams are not easy to buy—pharmacies just don't stock them. You can order them by asking your pharmacist to order them for you or by checking in the yellow pages under "Dental Equipment and Supplies." You can order them directly by mail from Cash and Carry in Hackensack, New Jersey. Call 201-487-4472.

Analingus (oral sex performed on the anus), sometimes called rimming, is considered by health experts to be unsafe, especially because diseases such as intestinal parasites and hepatitis can be spread. A dental dam may reduce the risk.

## A FINAL NOTE

We hope our suggestions will make it easier for you to persuade your lover to use a condom. That *you* want to use a condom is an important first step. You are acting wisely and responsibly, and we urge you to remember that if your partner tries to change your mind.

We've tried to be complete, but if you have questions that weren't answered in this book, or if you still have doubts, please don't hesitate to consult your doctor or call a local sex information line or the public health department. At the back of this book, we've listed some phone numbers that might be useful if you do have further questions.

# RESOURCE
# DIRECTORY

Following are the phone numbers of some information lines you can call if you want to find out more about AIDS, sexually transmitted diseases, condom use, or safe sex. In addition, many cities have local numbers for public health departments, sex information lines, crisis hotlines, VD clinics, and AIDS centers. You can usually find these numbers by calling your city or county public health department or mental health department, crisis or suicide intervention line, large church or synagogue, or telephone information. These can usually refer you to the organization that can answer your questions.

If you would like information about confidential testing for the AIDS virus, call your local or state health department.

Information on contraception is available from your local Planned Parenthood office. Consult your phone book or call directory assistance for the phone number of the Planned Parenthood office in your city. Or call the national Planned Parenthood office toll free at (800)

223-3303, or write to it: Planned Parenthood Federation of America, 810 Seventh Avenue, New York, NY 10019.

NATIONAL AIDS HOTLINE: (800) 342-2437 toll free, for recorded information about AIDS; (800) 443-0366 toll free, if you have specific questions

NATIONAL SEXUALLY TRANSMITTED DISEASES HOTLINE: (800) 227-8922

NATIONAL GAY TASK FORCE AIDS INFORMATION HOTLINE: (800) 221-7044; (212) 807-6016 (within New York state)

AMERICAN RED CROSS AIDS EDUCATION OFFICE: (202) 737-8300

SAN FRANCISCO AIDS HOTLINE: (415) 863-AIDS

SAN FRANCISCO SEX INFORMATION LINE: (415) 621-7300

NEW YORK GAY MEN'S HEALTH CRISIS INFORMATION LINE: (212) 807-6655

CHICAGO AIDS HOTLINE: (312) 871-5696

LOS ANGELES AIDS PROJECT HOTLINE: (213) 871-AIDS

MIAMI AIDS HOTLINE: (305) 634-4636

NEW ORLEANS AIDS EDUCATION HOTLINE:
(504) 522-2437

BOSTON AIDS ACTION LINE: (617) 536-7733

ATLANTA AIDS INFO LINE: (404) 876-9944;
(800) 551-2728 (toll free in Georgia)

MINNEAPOLIS AIDS HOTLINE: (612) 870-0700

# ABOUT THE
# AUTHORS

*Patti Breitman* is a book editor who has worked on several books in the health field, including *The AIDS Epidemic* by James Slaff, M.D., and John Brubaker (Warner Books, 1986).

*Kim Knutson* is a recent graduate from Harvard University. She holds a degree in psychology and is currently a publicist and book editor.

*Paul Reed* is a writer whose novel *Facing It* (Gay Sunshine Press, 1984) is the only novel yet published with AIDS as its central theme. Mr. Reed writes extensively on health issues and safe sexual practices and regularly contributes book reviews to the *Bay Area Reporter* and the *San Francisco Chronicle*. He holds a Master of Arts degree in anthropology from the University of California, Davis.

*John Money, Ph.D.*, is one of the nation's most respected and often quoted experts in the field of human sexuality.

He is a professor of medical psychology and pediatrics, emeritus at the John Hopkins University and Hospital. Dr. Money has written more than a dozen books for the scientific community and the general reader. He is also the author of more than 300 scientific papers and 75 scholarly reviews and textbook chapters.

This book is available at bulk discounts from the publisher. Schools, corporations, libraries, and medical centers can call the publisher for ordering information:

PRIMA PUBLISHING
AND COMMUNICATIONS
(916) 624-5718

## HOW TO ORDER:

Quantity discounts are available from Prima Publishing & Communications, Post Office Box 1260PC, Rocklin, CA 95677; Telephone: (916) 624-5718. On your letterhead, include information concerning the intended use of the books and the number of books you wish to purchase.